Sensei Self Development

Mental Health Chronicles Series

Identifying and Managing Unhealthy Habits

Sensei Paul David

Copyright Page

Sensei Self Development -
Identifying and Managing Unhealthy Habits,
by Sensei Paul David

Copyright © 2024

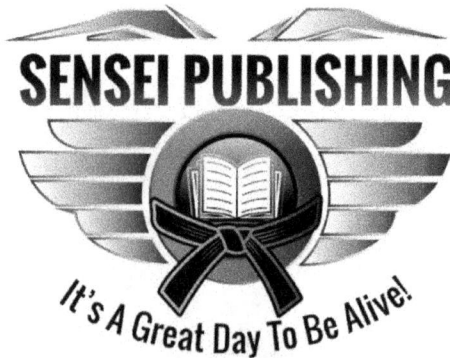

SENSEI PUBLISHING

It's A Great Day To Be Alive!

www.senseipublishing.com

@senseipublishing
#senseipublishing

Get/Share Your FREE SSD Mental Health Chronicles at

www.senseiselfdevelopment.care

or

CLICK HERE

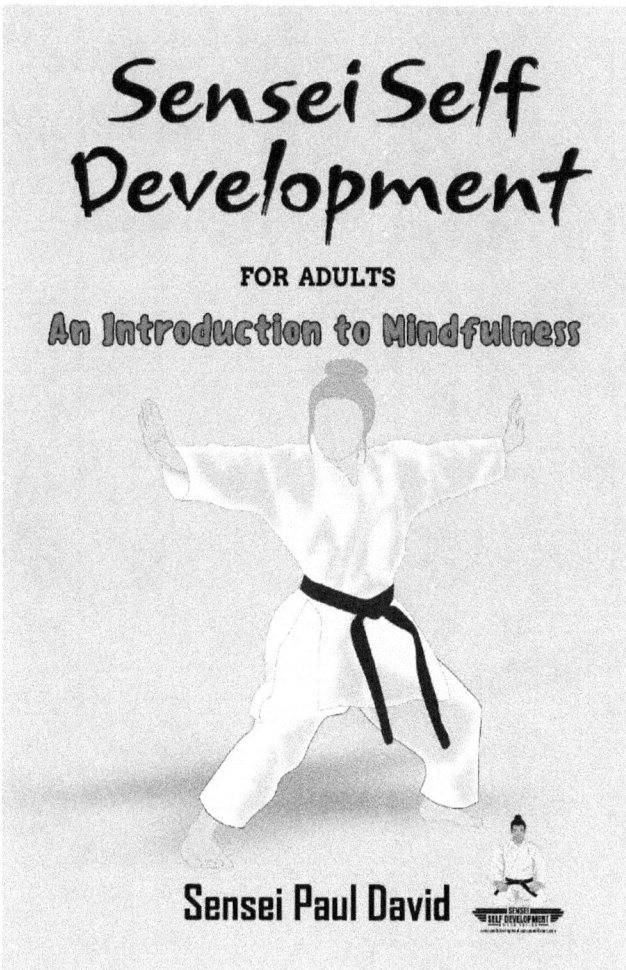

Check Out The SSD Chronicles Series CLICK HERE

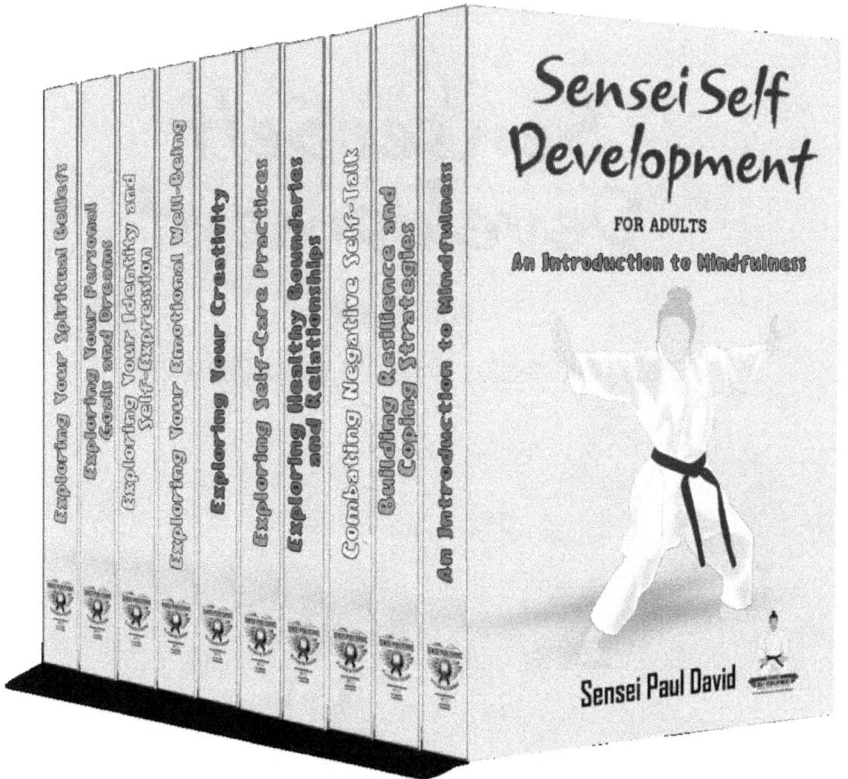

Exploring Your Spiritual Beliefs

Exploring Your Personal Goals and Dreams

Exploring Your Identity and Self-Expression

Exploring Your Emotional Well-Being

Exploring Your Creativity

Exploring Self-Care Practices

Exploring Healthy Boundaries and Relationships

Combatting Negative Self-Talk

Building Resilience and Coping Strategies

An Introduction to Mindfulness

Sensei Self Development

FOR ADULTS

An Introduction to Mindfulness

Sensei Paul David

Dedication

To those who courageously take action
towards self-improvement - you are helping to
evolve the world for generations to come.

- It's a great day to be alive!

If Found Please Contact:

_____

Reward If Found:

_____

MY
COMMITMENT

I, _____

commit to writing This Sensei Self Development Journal for at least 10 days in a row, starting: _____

Writing this journal is valuable to me because:

_____

_____

_____

_____

_____

_____

If I finish a minimum of 10 consecutive days of writing in this journal, I will reward myself by:

_____

_____

_____

_____

_____

_____

If I don't finish 10 days of writing this journal, I will promise to:

_____

_____

_____

_____

_____

_____

I will do the following things to ensure that I write in my Sensei Self Development Journal every day:

_____

_____

_____

_____

_____

_____

Get/Share Your FREE All-Ages Mental Health eBook Now at

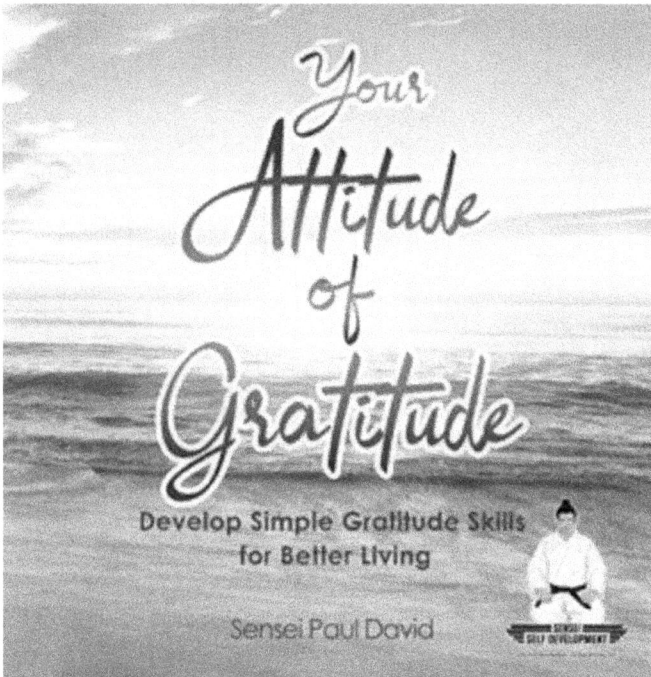

www.senseiselfdevelopment.com

Or CLICK HERE

Check Out Another Book In The
SSD BOOK SERIES:

CLICK HERE

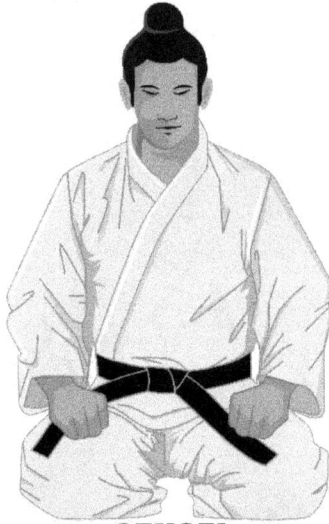

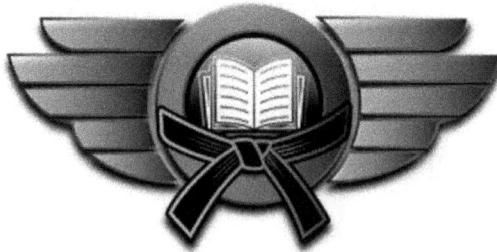

Join Our Publishing Journey!

If you would like to receive FUTURE FREE BOOKS and get to know us better, please click www.senseipublishing.com and join our newsletter by entering your email address in the pop-up box.

Follow Our Blog: senseipauldavid.ca

Follow/Like/Subscribe: Facebook, Instagram, YouTube: @senseipublishing

Scan the QR Code with your phone or tablet

to follow us on social media: Like / Subscribe / Follow

A Message From The Author:
Sensei Paul David

Dear Reader,

Welcome to the world of mental health journaling – a sacred space for self-reflection, growth, and healing. Within these pages, you hold the power to uplift your spirit, invigorate your mind, and nourish your goals.

In a world that often moves at blink-and-you'll-miss-it speed, it's crucial to make time for self-care and self-discovery.

Anxiety, stress, and emotional turbulence may have clouded your mind, making it difficult to find clarity and peace within. But fear not! Together, we will navigate the labyrinth of emotions, and experiences, helping to simplify the path to mental well-being.

This journal is not merely a bunch of blank pages awaiting your words. It is your compassionate companion, offering solace and understanding during your unique journey. Here, you are free to unburden yourself, celebrate small and large victories, and confront the challenges that may still linger.

Within the sheltered realm of these pages, there is no judgment, no expectation, and no pressure. Your unique experience and perspective hold immeasurable worth, and your voice deserves to be heard. Whether you choose to fill the lines with eloquence or simply scribble fragments of your thoughts, please remember each entry is a valuable contribution to your growth.

In this sacred space, you are challenged to take off the mask we so often wear in the outside world. It is here that you can be raw, vulnerable, and authentic – allowing your true self to be seen and embraced without reservation. By giving yourself permission to explore the depths of your emotions and confront the shadows that may lurk within, you will discover profound insights and find the healing you seek over time.

As you embark on this journaling journey, I encourage you to embrace the process itself rather than fixate solely on the outcome. Remember, it is not about reaching a certain destination or ticking off boxes on a list of accomplishments. Rather, it is about cultivating self-awareness, fostering self-compassion, and nurturing a sense of curiosity about the intricate workings of your intelligently beautiful mind.

In the quiet moments of reflection, let your pen become a bridge between your inner world and the possibilities that lie ahead. Create a sanctuary for your thoughts, fears, triumphs, and dreams. As you pour your heart onto these pages, allow your words to be a living testament to courage, resilience, and an unwavering commitment to your own well-being.

I am honored to be a part of your journey, and I believe in your ability to navigate the twists and turns with grace and resilience. Remember, you are not alone in this – countless others have walked similar paths, faced similar challenges, and emerged stronger and wiser on the other side. You have the power to reclaim all of your untapped joy, cultivate a positive mindset that serves you, and foster a deep sense of self-love and peaceful confident. – And it will take a worth effort and time.

So, open the first page of this journal with hope, curiosity, and an open heart and open mind. Embrace the transformative power of self-reflection, and allow it to guide you towards a life of greater fulfilment and peace. Each journaling session is an opportunity to not only connect with yourself but also to rekindle the light within that sometimes flickers but never extinguishes.

Remember, the pages you are about to fill are not just a record of your journey but also a testament to your strength, resilience, and indomitable spirit. Cherish this space, invest in yourself, and let your words be an ode to the magnificent journey of becoming whole.

With great respect for your decision to evolve,

Paul

MY CONVICTION

Please circle your answers below

I am DECIDING to be patient with myself and this PROCESS each time I journal toward my improved state of mental well-being

YES   NO

"The present moment is filled with joy and
happiness. If you are attentive,
you will see it."

Thich Nhat Hanh

Introduction

Understanding why we can't easily stop unhealthy habits, despite knowing their negative effects, is complex. A large number of smokers, for example, express a desire to quit, yet find it extremely difficult. This struggle is similar for those dealing with drug and alcohol addictions, which can have devastating effects on both health and personal relationships. Even in cases of excess weight, where the benefits of a healthy diet and exercise are well-known, making these lifestyle changes can be a real challenge.

The difficulty in breaking unhealthy habits and making positive changes is deeply rooted in how our brains work. Habits, both good and bad, form neural pathways in the brain, making them entrenched and automatic responses to certain stimuli or situations. Once these pathways are established, they can be incredibly hard to alter or break.

The key to understanding this lies in the neuroscience of habit formation. Studies have shown that habits are more than just repeated behaviors; they are complex processes involving different parts of the brain. These processes involve the creation of a routine that, once triggered by a cue, can almost run automatically.

This understanding has led to the development of strategies aimed at breaking these patterns. Instead of just trying to stop a behavior, the focus is on altering the underlying cognitive and neurological pathways. This might involve creating new habits that replace the old ones, changing the environment to remove cues that trigger the behavior, or using techniques that target the brain's reward system to diminish the appeal of the bad habit.

Changing deeply ingrained habits requires more than just willpower; it requires a comprehensive understanding of the cognitive and neurological aspects of these behaviors.

By approaching habit change from this angle, there's a greater chance of making lasting changes.

Habits are not all bad as we know. They are formed through repetition and are a natural, often beneficial part of our lives. Consider the daily routines we perform without conscious thought, like showering, combing hair, or brushing teeth. These habits save mental energy, allowing the brain to focus on other tasks. Similarly, driving on familiar routes can happen almost automatically, thanks to these ingrained habits.

However, we are all too well aware that not all habits are beneficial. The brain's reward centers can be triggered by pleasurable experiences, leading to potentially harmful routines. This is evident in behaviors like overeating, smoking, drug or alcohol abuse, gambling, and even compulsive use of computers and social media.

The process of forming these habits, whether beneficial or harmful, involves the same underlying brain mechanisms. This means that the brain structure that helps us perform routine tasks without thinking is the same one that can lead to detrimental habits. This similarity in how different types of habits are formed highlights the complexity of our brain functions and the challenges involved in managing our behaviors.

But there's a crucial difference in how pleasure-based habits are formed that makes them harder to break. When we engage in enjoyable activities, our brain releases dopamine, a chemical that reinforces the pleasure and satisfaction we feel. This dopamine release strengthens the habit every time we engage in the activity. It also creates a craving when we're not indulging in the behavior. This is why some individuals might crave drugs even if they no longer provide a pleasurable feeling.

This mechanism means that in many cases, our brains can work against us when we try to overcome bad habits. These habits can become deeply ingrained, almost hardwired into our brains. The reward centers continue to drive cravings for the very things we are attempting to avoid.

But there is reason to be hopeful. Humans aren't just creatures of habit; we have other brain regions that assist us in making decisions that are beneficial for our health and can work to counteract our bad behaviors.

Causes of Unhealthy Habits

Bad habits typically stem from two main sources: stress and boredom. When we feel stressed or bored, we often turn to certain behaviors as a quick way to alleviate these feelings. This could be anything from nail-biting in moments of anxiety, to going on a shopping spree for a dopamine rush, indulging in alcohol during the weekends to unwind, or endlessly scrolling through the internet to fill time.

However, these habits are not the only way to deal with stress and boredom. It's possible to cultivate healthier alternatives. For instance, instead of spending hours online, one might choose to go for a run, start a creative project, or practice meditation. These healthier activities provide a more constructive way to manage stress and boredom.

That said, the apparent stress or boredom might just be the tip of the iceberg, often masking deeper, more complex issues. It could be deeply ingrained beliefs, unresolved events from the past, or underlying fears that drive these habits. Tackling these deeper issues requires honesty and self-reflection. It's about asking hard questions: What beliefs are fueling these habits? Is there a fear or past event that's holding me back?

Fast Facts

1. Neuroplasticity and Habits: The brain's ability to rewire itself, known as neuroplasticity, plays a crucial role in breaking habits. Forming new

habits actually changes the structure of the brain.

2. Dopamine's Double-Edged Sword: While dopamine release is associated with pleasure and reinforces habits, it's also released as a response to novelty. This means introducing new, positive activities can leverage dopamine's effects to break bad habits.

3. The 21-Day Myth: The common belief that it takes 21 days to form or break a habit is a myth. Studies suggest it can take anywhere from 18 to 254 days, depending on the individual and the habit.

4. Emotional Connection: Emotional states significantly influence habits. Stress and negative emotions can strengthen bad habits, while positive emotions can help in forming good habits.

5. The Role of Environment: Environmental cues often trigger habits. Changing your

environment can be a powerful way to break bad habits and form new ones.

6. Social Influence: People are more likely to succeed in breaking habits if they are surrounded by others who support their goals or share similar aspirations.

7. Small Changes, Big Impact: Breaking a habit doesn't always require massive changes. Small, incremental adjustments can lead to significant long-term habit change.

8. Mindfulness and Awareness: Mindfulness practices can increase awareness of habit triggers and automatic responses, giving an opportunity to choose different actions.

9. The Power of Habit Stacking: Adding a new habit onto an existing one, known as habit stacking, can make it easier to adopt the new habit.

10. Failure as Part of the Process: Failing to stick to new habits is often part of the journey. Each attempt at breaking a habit can be a learning experience, contributing to eventual success.

How to Break Unhealthy Habits

Lower Your Stress Levels and Fix Your Lifestyle

Many bad habits, such as smoking or excessive sugar intake, are closely linked to the brain's dopamine system. Dopamine, a chemical that creates a sense of pleasure, is released during rewarding activities. The first time you try a rewarding behavior, the rush of dopamine can lead to a euphoric feeling. This dopamine release not only affects the connections between neurons but also impacts the brain systems that govern our actions, playing a significant role in the formation of bad habits.

The allure of these stimuli, like sugar or certain substances, is very strong, and our response to them is deeply rooted in our evolutionary history. In prehistoric times, food wasn't processed or flavored as it is today. Our brains aren't fully equipped to handle the intense pleasure that modern, highly stimulating substances can provide. As a result, the frontal lobe, which acts as the brain's control center, can become overwhelmed.

To resist any kind of craving or temptation you need willpower, which is greatly reduced or depleted when you are under stress. So, to be able to break these habits you must have your power level at least halfway decent. You might have noticed it is hard to force yourself to do something when you are sleep-deprived or when you are tired. You get irritated quicker and lash out. You find it harder to resist junk food. That's because you are low on willpower. Something similar happens under stress.

To counteract these tendencies, incorporating lifestyle changes like getting sufficient sleep, exercising regularly, and practicing stress-reduction techniques such as meditation can be beneficial. These activities lower stress levels, help bolster willpower, and improve overall brain health, making it easier to resist the pull of bad habits.

Identify Your Cues

Habits typically consist of three elements: a cue, a routine, and a reward. Cues are specific contexts or situations that trigger the habit. For instance, a smoker might associate taking work breaks with smoking, or a dessert lover might find the mere act of looking at a dessert menu triggering.

Understanding these cues or triggers is crucial for managing habits. For smokers, it might be helpful to remove items like ashtrays that remind them of smoking. Similarly, those trying to reduce alcohol consumption should consider avoiding routes that pass by their favorite bar.

Significant life changes, like moving to a new city or starting a new job, can provide an excellent opportunity to break bad habits. These changes bring new contexts and situations, devoid of the usual cues, making it easier to form new, healthier habits. For example, a smoker relocating to a new city might use the opportunity to change their commute, engaging in different activities like public transportation or listening to a new podcast, instead of smoking. This change in environment can be a strategic advantage in breaking the cycle of an established habit.

But you don't have to move to a new city, simply identifying your cue can help tremendously.

Replace A Bad Habit With A Good

Replacing a bad habit with a good one can be more effective than trying to simply stop a behavior. We are inherently action-oriented, and research shows that suppressing thoughts often leads to a rebound effect. For example, studies have found that people trying to suppress thoughts about eating chocolate ended up consuming more, and smokers who tried to restrain thoughts about smoking thought about it even more.

Instead of telling yourself not to engage in a bad habit, it's more effective to replace it with a positive action. If you're trying to quit smoking, for instance, try chewing gum whenever the urge to smoke arises. If your routine involves having a glass of wine at 5 p.m., consider replacing it with a healthy habit like drinking flavored seltzer or cold water with lemon.

It's important to remember that forming a new habit takes time and commitment. Research has indicated that it can take an average of 66 days for a behavior to become habitual, though the time can vary greatly. So, patience and persistence are key when trying to establish new, healthier routines in place of old habits.

Find the Reason Why You Want to Change

Even if you substitute a negative habit with a better one, the original habit might still offer a stronger biological reward. For example, substituting sugary snacks with fruit may not provide the same immediate pleasure rush due to lower sugar levels. This is why having strong personal motivation is key.

We might understand the general benefits of certain changes, like reducing sugar intake for better health or exercising more for weight management. However, tying these habit changes to specific, personal goals can be more motivating. For instance, cutting back on sugar might be motivated by the goal of improving energy levels for daily activities, or regular exercise could be about training for a specific event or challenge. These personalized motivations can be a powerful driving force, especially when the biological rewards of the less healthy habits are more immediately satisfying.

Introduce Friction

Transforming a negative behavior into a positive one can be achieved by adding a layer of difficulty or inconvenience, a strategy known as adding friction. This concept is well-demonstrated in behavioral studies. For instance, one classic study in the Journal of Applied Behaviour Analysis explored how to encourage people to choose stairs over an elevator. Researchers in a four-story building increased the time it took for the elevator doors to close by 16 seconds. This seemingly minor inconvenience significantly reduced elevator usage by one-third. What's remarkable is that even after the elevator speed was returned to normal, many people continued to prefer the stairs, having developed a new habit of stair-climbing.

Similarly, if you're trying to reduce prolonged sitting at a computer, switching to a hard-backed chair can make sitting for long periods uncomfortable. This discomfort encourages more frequent standing breaks, thereby reducing the habit of constant sitting.

The key to adding friction is creating a slight but noticeable barrier that disrupts the automatic nature of the habit. This small change in the environment or routine can be enough to pause and reconsider the action, allowing for the opportunity to replace it with a more positive behavior. Over time, this conscious effort can turn into a new, healthier habit, as the brain starts to associate the new behavior with the specific context or cue. This method effectively leverages our innate preference for ease and comfort to foster better habits.

Find a Partner

When trying to break an unwanted habit, having a friend or partner join you in the effort can be incredibly beneficial. For instance, if you both want to quit smoking, facing the challenge together can make a big difference. While teaming up won't eliminate the cravings, dealing with them can become more manageable when you're not doing it alone.

It's important to actively support each other. Celebrating each other's successes and offering encouragement during tough times strengthens your resolve and maintains motivation. This shared journey creates a sense of accountability and camaraderie, making the process less daunting.

Even if your friend doesn't have a habit they're trying to change, their support can still be invaluable. Letting a trusted friend know about your goal to break a habit allows them to offer encouragement and keep you focused. They can be a source of motivation during moments of doubt and can gently nudge you back on track if they see you reverting to old patterns. This external support system can be a key factor in successfully overcoming challenging habits.

Use Visualization

Visualizing yourself successfully overcoming a habit in a triggering situation can be a powerful tool.

For example, picture yourself on a stressful morning, perhaps before a performance review. Think about your typical response in such a scenario. Maybe you'd find yourself biting your nails or tapping your pen on the desk.

Now, reimagine that situation with a positive twist. Visualize yourself engaging in calming activities instead. Perhaps you see yourself taking deep breaths, getting up to drink some water, going through old notes or files, or organizing your desk drawers. These alternative actions keep your hands occupied and help soothe your nerves.

This mental rehearsal is about preparing yourself to respond differently in situations that usually trigger the unwanted habit. By vividly imagining yourself performing a different, more positive action, you're mentally paving the way for actual behavioral change. This practice can reinforce your real-life efforts to break the habit, making it easier to respond in healthier ways when the actual situation arises.

Alter Your Reward and Punishment Matrix

Being aware of your actions in real-time can play a significant role in changing ingrained habits. Next time you find yourself procrastinating or reaching the end of a large bag of snacks, take a moment to reflect on what you're feeling. Ask yourself what you're gaining from this action. This mindfulness approach can be quite effective in altering habitual behavior.

For instance, in a study involving over 1,000 patients who had a habit of overeating, the participants were encouraged to really focus on how they felt during binge eating sessions. By consciously observing their feelings and behaviors during these episodes 10 to 15 times, they began to notice a decrease in their urge to overindulge. They also reported a significant reduction in craving-driven eating. As they became more aware that their habitual behavior wasn't beneficial, the rewarding feeling they previously associated with it diminished. They effectively became disenchanted with their old behavior.

Another mindful strategy is to think about how much better you feel when you don't engage in your bad habit. Our brain is constantly seeking a 'bigger, better offer' (BBO). If you can concentrate on how unrewarding your old behavior is compared to how rewarding a new behavior could be, your brain will naturally gravitate towards the latter. For example, instead of spending excessive time on social media, engaging in meaningful conversations with friends can be your BBO. Or, choosing to go for a morning run might give you an all-day high, in contrast to the regret you might feel for skipping it. This focus on the positive outcomes of changing your behavior can significantly influence your brain's decision-making process, steering it towards healthier habits.

Have a Backup for Your Backup

What if you try to replace your bad habit with a good habit but you still feel tempted?

In moments of temptation, it's useful to have a primary backup plan and a secondary, more indulgent, backup plan. The primary plan offers a healthier alternative, while the secondary plan is slightly more indulgent but still better than the original bad habit.

For example, if you're trying to cut down on alcohol, your primary plan might be to choose sparkling water. However, if the craving persists and sparkling water doesn't suffice, your secondary backup plan could be to have a small glass of soda. This secondary option is more indulgent compared to sparkling water, but it's still a better choice than alcohol.

Having a secondary backup plan that's a bit more gratifying can make the transition away from a bad habit more manageable. It acts as a middle ground, offering some level of satisfaction without fully reverting to the old, unhealthy habit.

This two-tiered approach helps in managing cravings or moments of weakness more effectively. Over time, as you get more accustomed to healthier choices, you may find that your reliance on the secondary, more indulgent backup plan decreases. The key is gradual progress and flexibility, allowing for a balance between discipline and indulgence as you work to replace bad habits with healthier ones.

Keep Self Compassion in Mind

Changing habits is a journey full of ups and downs, and it's crucial to accept that progress isn't always a straight line. Setbacks and challenges are a normal part of making lasting changes. Often, we tend to be our own harshest critics, thinking that anything short of complete success is a total failure.

Imagine how you would respond to a friend who slips up on their diet by having a bag of chips. You'd likely be supportive and understanding, not overly critical. It's important to extend this same kindness and reassurance to yourself. Recognize that self-critical thoughts are just thoughts; they don't reflect reality. Like in meditation, the idea is to notice these thoughts without getting caught up in them, letting them pass through your mind without judgment.

Remember that the goal isn't to completely eliminate the old habit overnight. It's more about gradually building up the new, healthier habit so that it becomes stronger and more prevalent. Knowing that the old habit won't just vanish can ease the pressure and feelings of failure.

Life is unpredictable and full of surprises, and you can't always foresee every trigger or challenge. Approaching these situations with self-compassion and understanding that habit change is an ongoing process can make it more achievable. Being gentle with yourself, acknowledging that setbacks are part of the journey, and focusing on strengthening new habits can lead to more sustainable and meaningful changes.

A Personal Anecdote: How I Fought My Phone Addiction

To fight my phone addiction, I first had to admit I was dependent on it and see how it was negatively affecting my work, social interactions, and even my driving. I then focused on what specifically triggered my urge to check my phone. For me, these triggers were the sounds – like notification pings – and the visuals, such as pop-up notifications.

Simply silencing my phone wasn't enough. Inspired by the marshmallow experiment, I realized that keeping my phone out of sight could help. So, in the morning while making breakfast, I left it in a different room. When driving, I stowed it away in the glove compartment, and while walking, I put it in a zippered pocket.

I found that adding friction was effective. Completely turning off my phone worked better than just silencing it. The deterrent wasn't my curiosity about messages; it was the inconvenience of turning the phone back on.

I also looked for new rewards to replace the gratification I got from my phone. In the car, I switched to listening to the radio. In the evenings, instead of scrolling through social media, I discovered new authors to read.

These alternatives genuinely enriched my life and made me feel calmer and more liberated at the end of the day. Breaking free from my phone addiction became a real, achievable goal.

Before We Get Started…

Remember, mindfulness journaling is a personal practice, and these questions are meant to guide and inspire you. Feel free to adapt and modify them to suit your needs and preferences. Explore, reflect, and embrace the opportunity to deepen your self-awareness and cultivate a sense of inner peace.

Date ___ / ___ / ___: S   M   T   W   Th   F   S

I feel:
(please circle)

because   because   because   because   because
_____ _____ _____ _____ _____
_____ _____ _____ _____ _____

Today I Am Grateful For

1. _____
2. _____
3. _____

What could help transform today into a remarkable day?

Reflective Writing

How do unhealthy habits manifest themselves in my life?

_____

_____

_____

_____

_____

_____

_____

Which of the following is NOT an unhealthy habit?

a) Stress eating
b) Exercising regularly
c) Smoking
d) Binge-watching TV shows

All Are Correct - Choose The Response You Feel Is Most Important To Remember

Date ___ / ___ / ___: **S   M   T   W   Th   F   S**

I feel:
(please circle)

because _____
because _____
because _____
because _____
because _____

Today I Am Grateful For

1. _____
2. _____
3. _____

What could help transform today into a remarkable day?

Reflective Writing

How have my unhealthy habits affected my relationships with others?

_____

_____

_____

_____

_____

_____

_____

Which of the following is a potential consequence of an unhealthy habit?

a) Improved cardiovascular health
b) Increased energy levels
c) Poor mental health
d) Stronger immune system

All Are Correct - Choose The Response You Feel Is Most Important To Remember

Date ___ / ___ / ___ : S   M   T   W   Th   F   S

I feel:
(please circle)

because _____   because _____   because _____   because _____   because _____

Today I Am Grateful For

1. _____
2. _____
3. _____

What could help transform today into a remarkable day?

Reflective Writing

What steps can I take to become aware of my own unhealthy habits?

_____

_____

_____

_____

_____

_____

_____

Which of the following is an example of an unhealthy habit related to nutrition?

a) Eating a balanced diet
b) Skipping meals
c) Drinking plenty of water
d) Avoiding processed foods

All Are Correct - Choose The Response You Feel Is Most Important To Remember

Date ___ / ___ / ___ : S M T W Th F S

I feel:
(please circle)

because   because   because   because   because

_____ _____ _____ _____ _____

_____ _____ _____ _____ _____

Today I Am Grateful For

1. _____
2. _____
3. _____

What could help transform today into a remarkable day?

Reflective Writing

What strategies can I use to begin to manage my
unhealthy habits?

_____

_____

_____

_____

_____

_____

_____

_____

Which of the following is NOT a way to manage and break an unhealthy habit?

a) Setting realistic goals
b) Ignoring the habit completely
c) Developing a support system
d) Seeking professional help

All Are Correct - Choose The Response You Feel Is Most Important To Remember

Date ___ / ___ / ___: S M T W Th F S

I feel:
(please circle)

because because because because because

_____ _____ _____ _____ _____

_____ _____ _____ _____ _____

Today I Am Grateful For

1. _____
2. _____
3. _____

What could help transform today into a remarkable day?

Reflective Writing

What can I do to help motivate
myself to make changes?

_____

_____

_____

_____

_____

_____

_____

Which of the following is an unhealthy habit related to sleep?

a) Getting 8 hours of rest each night
b) Staying up late to finish tasks
c) Taking regular naps
d) Establishing a bedtime routine

All Are Correct - Choose The Response You Feel Is Most Important To Remember

Date ___ / ___ / ___ : S M T W Th F S

I feel: 😊 😁 😋 😣 😠
(please circle) because because because because because
_____ _____ _____ _____ _____
_____ _____ _____ _____ _____

Today I Am Grateful For

1. _____
2. _____
3. _____

What could help transform today into a remarkable day?

Reflective Writing

How can I create an environment where I
am more likely to make healthier choices?

_____

_____

_____

_____

_____

_____

_____

Which of the following is an example of an unhealthy habit related to stress management?

a) Meditation and deep breathing
b) Exercising regularly
c) Engaging in unhealthy coping mechanisms
d) Taking breaks throughout the day

All Are Correct - Choose The Response You Feel Is Most Important To Remember

Date ___ / ___ / ___: S M T W Th F S

I feel:
(please circle)

because   because   because   because   because
_____ _____ _____ _____ _____
_____ _____ _____ _____ _____

Today I Am Grateful For

1. _____
2. _____
3. _____

What could help transform today into a remarkable day?

Reflective Writing

What are the consequences of unhealthy habits
and how can I avoid them?

_____

_____

_____

_____

_____

_____

_____

Which of the following is an unhealthy habit related to physical activity?

a) Regular exercise routine
b) Being sedentary for long periods of time
c) Participating in team sports
d) Taking frequent walks throughout the day

All Are Correct - Choose The Response You Feel Is Most Important To Remember

Date ___ / ___ / ___: S M T W Th F S

I feel:
(please circle)

because _____
because _____
because _____
because _____
because _____

Today I Am Grateful For

1. _____
2. _____
3. _____

What could help transform today into a remarkable day?

Reflective Writing

How can I set realistic goals to
make healthy changes?

_____

_____

_____

_____

_____

_____

Which of the following is NOT a strategy for identifying and managing unhealthy habits?

a) Keeping a journal
b) Seeking advice from friends and family
c) Self-reflection and introspection
d) Denying the existence of unhealthy habits

All Are Correct - Choose The Response You Feel Is Most Important To Remember

Date ___ / ___ / ___ : **S   M   T   W   Th   F   S**

I feel:
(please circle)

because _____ because _____ because _____ because _____ because _____
_____ _____ _____ _____ _____

Today I Am Grateful For

1. _____
2. _____
3. _____

What could help transform today into a remarkable day?

Reflective Writing

What tools can I use to track my progress in managing my unhealthy habits?

_____

_____

_____

_____

_____

_____

_____

Which of the following is an example of an unhealthy habit related to technology use?

a) Setting limits on screen time
b) Constantly checking social media
c) Using technology for work or productivity
d) Prioritizing face-to-face interactions over online interactions

All Are Correct - Choose The Response You Feel Is Most Important To Remember

Date ___ / ___ / ___: S   M   T   W   Th   F   S

I feel:
(please circle)

because _____   because _____   because _____   because _____   because _____

Today I Am Grateful For

1. _____
2. _____
3. _____

What could help transform today into a remarkable day?

Reflective Writing

What can I do to help prevent the development of new unhealthy habits?

_____

_____

_____

_____

_____

_____

_____

Which of the following is a potential consequence of an unhealthy habit?

a) Improved memory and cognitive function
b) Decreased risk of chronic diseases
c) Increased stress and anxiety
d) Stronger relationships and social connections

All Are Correct - Choose The Response You Feel Is Most Important To Remember

47

Date ___ / ___ / ___ : S   M   T   W   Th   F   S

I feel:
(please circle)

because   because   because   because   because
_____ _____ _____ _____ _____
_____ _____ _____ _____ _____

Today I Am Grateful For

1. _____
2. _____
3. _____

What could help transform today into a remarkable day?

Reflective Writing

What are the benefits of managing my
unhealthy habits?

_____

_____

_____

_____

_____

_____

_____

Which of the following is an unhealthy habit related to alcohol consumption?

a) Drinking in moderation
b) Binge drinking
c) Drinking water in between alcoholic beverages
d) Experimenting with new types of alcohol

All Are Correct - Choose The Response You Feel Is Most Important To Remember

Date ___/___/___: S M T W Th F S

I feel:
(please circle)

because _____
because _____
because _____
because _____
because _____

Today I Am Grateful For

1. _____
2. _____
3. _____

What could help transform today into a remarkable day?

Reflective Writing
How can I find support and encouragement when trying to make changes?

_____
_____
_____
_____
_____
_____
_____

Which of the following is NOT a helpful approach to breaking an unhealthy habit?

a) Making excuses for the habit
b) Seeking support from friends and family
c) Replacing the habit with a healthier alternative
d) Setting specific and achievable goals

All Are Correct - Choose The Response You Feel Is Most Important To Remember

Date ___ / ___ / ___: S   M   T   W   Th   F   S

I feel:
(please circle)

because   because   because   because   because
_____ _____ _____ _____ _____
_____ _____ _____ _____ _____

Today I Am Grateful For

1. _____
2. _____
3. _____

What could help transform today into a remarkable day?

Reflective Writing

What techniques can I use to stay focused and
motivated when working on my unhealthy habits?

_____

_____

_____

_____

_____

_____

_____

_____

_____

Which of the following is an unhealthy habit related to self-care?

a) Practicing regular self-care routines
b) Neglecting personal hygiene
c) Taking breaks to relax and recharge
d) Engaging in activities that bring joy and fulfillment

All Are Correct - Choose The Response You Feel Is Most Important To Remember

Date ___ / ___ / ___ : S M T W Th F S

I feel:
(please circle)

because _____ _____

because _____ _____

because _____ _____

because _____ _____

because _____ _____

Today I Am Grateful For

1. _____
2. _____
3. _____

What could help transform today into a remarkable day?

Reflective Writing

How can I be kind to myself when I am struggling
with my unhealthy habits?

_____

_____

_____

_____

_____

_____

_____

Which of the following is NOT a potential consequence of an unhealthy habit?

a) Decreased risk of chronic diseases
b) Negative impact on mental health
c) Increased financial burden
d) Strained relationships with loved ones

All Are Correct - Choose The Response You Feel Is Most Important To Remember

Date ___ / ___ / ___ : S   M   T   W   Th   F   S

I feel: because   because   because   because   because
(please circle) _____   _____   _____   _____   _____
                 _____   _____   _____   _____   _____

Today I Am Grateful For

1. _____
2. _____
3. _____

What could help transform today into a remarkable day?

Reflective Writing

What can I do to ensure that I stay on track with
managing my unhealthy habits?

_____

_____

_____

_____

_____

_____

_____

Which of the following is an example of an unhealthy habit related to relationships?

a) Setting healthy boundaries in relationships

b) Ignoring red flags or warning signs in relationships

c) Actively listening and communicating in relationships

d) Investing time and effort into nurturing relationships

All Are Correct - Choose The Response You Feel Is Most Important To Remember

As we reach the final pages of this journey through "Positive Mindset," I want to extend my heartfelt thanks to you. Your commitment to exploring positivity and its transformative power is not only commendable but a testament to your desire for personal growth and a richer, more fulfilling life experience.

Remember, the journey towards a positive mindset is ongoing and ever-evolving. Each day presents new opportunities to apply these principles, to learn, and to grow. I encourage you to revisit these pages whenever you need a reminder of your incredible potential to foster positivity and resilience in the face of life's challenges.

As we part ways, I leave you with a quote that has been a guiding star in my journey: "The greatest discovery of any generation is that a human can alter his life by altering his attitude."

— William James.

Thank you for allowing me to be a part of your journey. May your path be filled with light, hope, and endless possibilities. Farewell, and may you carry the spirit of positivity with you, today and always.

With gratitude and best wishes,

Sensei Paul David

Reflective Writing

_____

_____

_____

_____

_____

_____

_____

_____

_____

_____

_____

_____

_____

_____

_____

_____

_____

_____

_____

_____

_____

_____

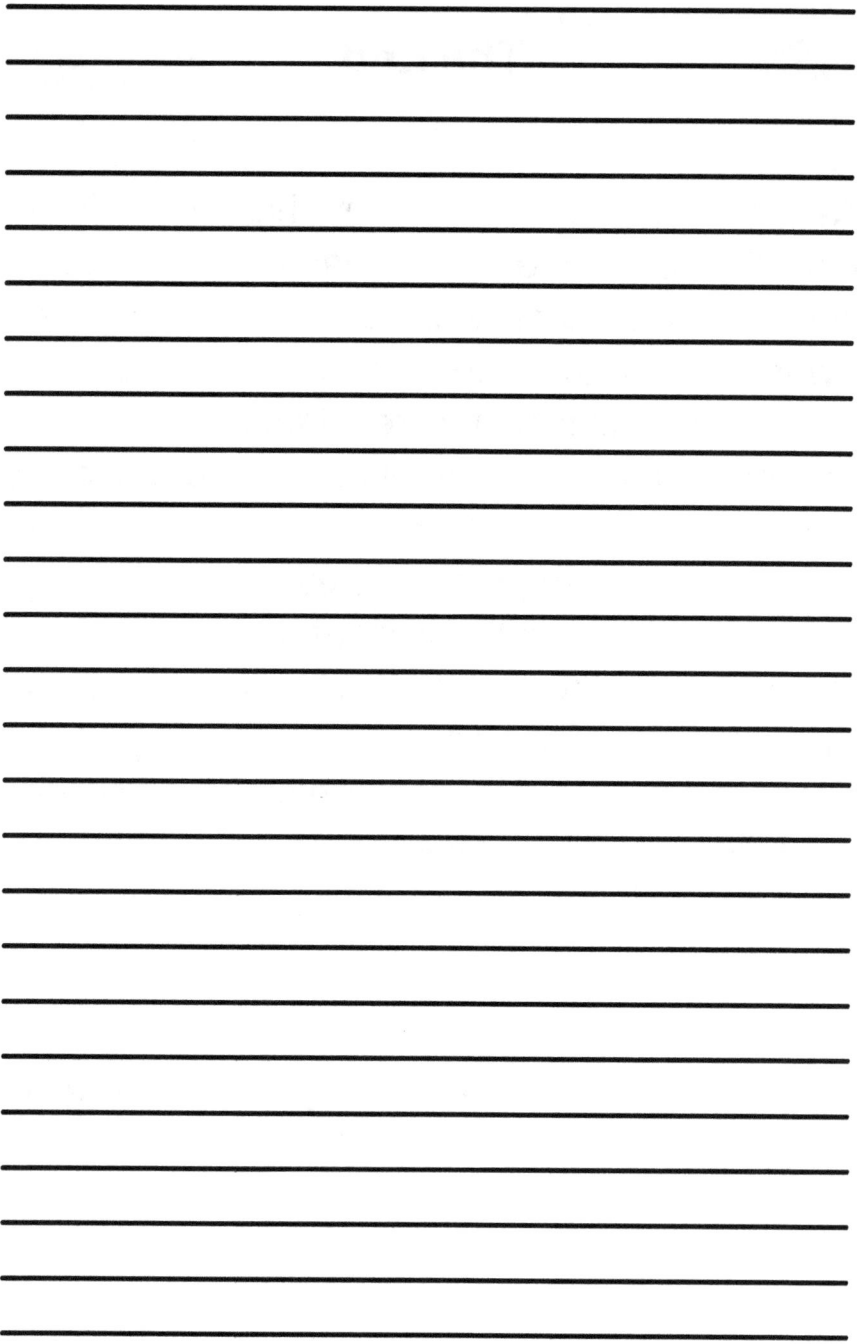

The End

As you close the pages of this mindfulness journal, remember that each word you've written is a step on your journey towards self-awareness and inner peace. Embrace the moments of clarity, the revelations, and even the uncertainties you've encountered along the way. Let this journal be a testament to your growth and a reminder that every day offers a new opportunity to be present, to observe, and to appreciate the simple wonders of life. Carry these lessons forward, and may your path be filled with mindful moments and serene reflections. Until we meet again in these pages, be gentle with yourself and stay anchored in the now.

Mindfulness isn't difficult, we just need to remember to do it.

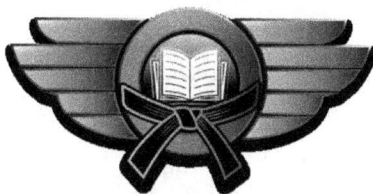

Thank You!

If you found this book helpful, I would be grateful if you would **post an honest review on Amazon** so this book can reach other supportive readers like you!

All you need to do is digitally flip to the back and leave your review. Or visit amazon.com/author/senseipauldavid click the correct book cover and click on the blue link next to the yellow stars that say, "customer reviews."

As always...
It's a great day to be alive!

Get/Share Your FREE SSD Mental Health Chronicles at
www.senseiselfdevelopment.care

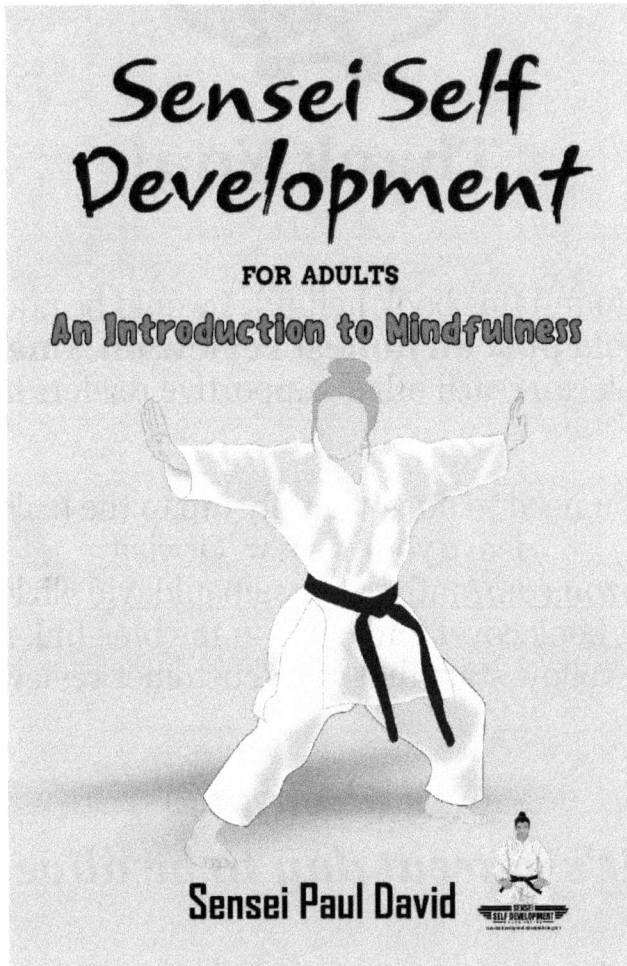

Sensei Self Development

FOR ADULTS

An Introduction to Mindfulness

Sensei Paul David

Check Out The SSD Chronicles
Series CLICK HERE

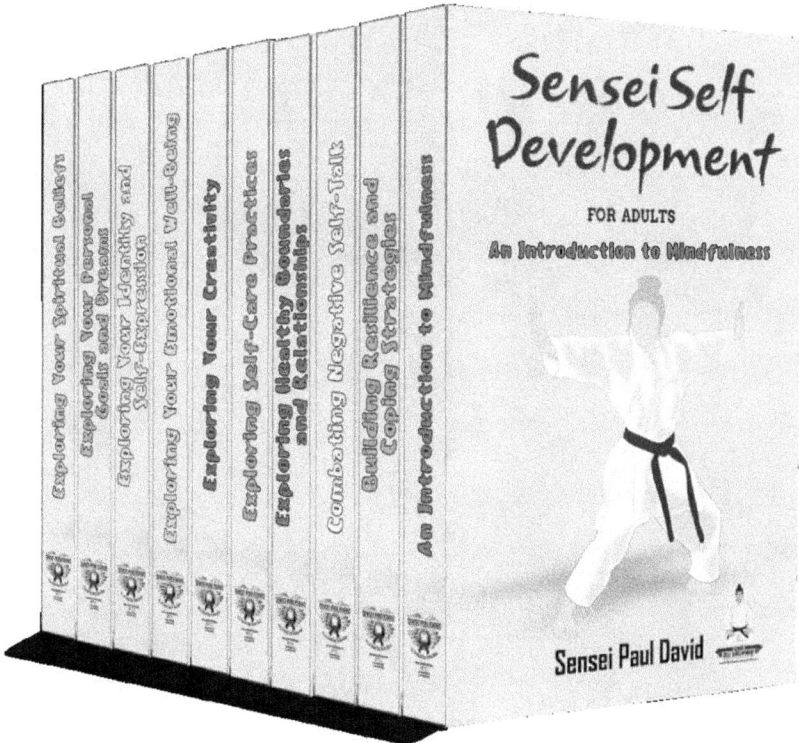

Exploring Your Spiritual Beliefs

Exploring Your Personal Goals and Dreams

Exploring Your Identity and Self-Expression

Exploring Your Emotional Well-Being

Exploring Your Creativity

Exploring Self-Care Practices

Exploring Healthy Boundaries and Relationships

Combating Negative Self-Talk

Building Resilience and Coping Strategies

An Introduction to Mindfulness

Sensei Self Development

FOR ADULTS

An Introduction to Mindfulness

Sensei Paul David

Get/Share Your FREE All-Ages Mental Health eBook Now at

www.senseiselfdevelopment.com

Or CLICK HERE

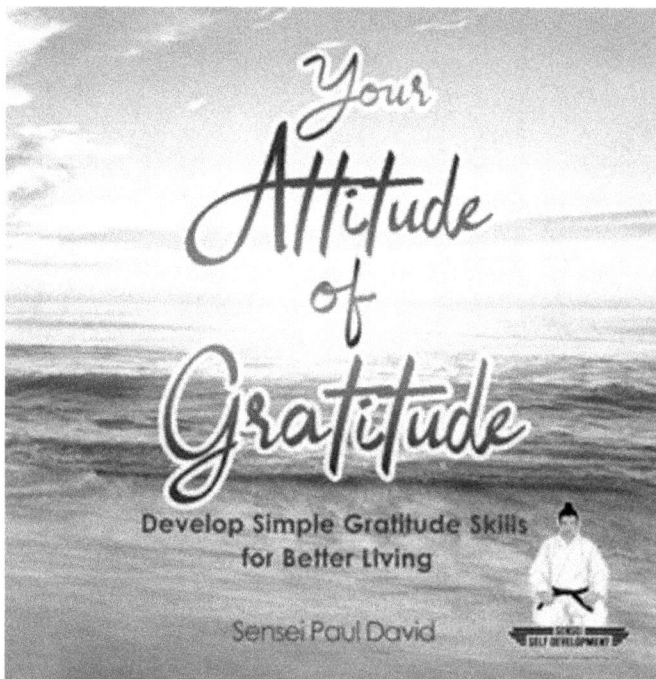

senseiselfdevelopment.com

Click Another Book In The SSD BOOK SERIES:

senseipublishing.com/SSD_SERIES

CLICK HERE

SENSEI
SELF DEVELOPMENT
— B O O K S S E R I E S —

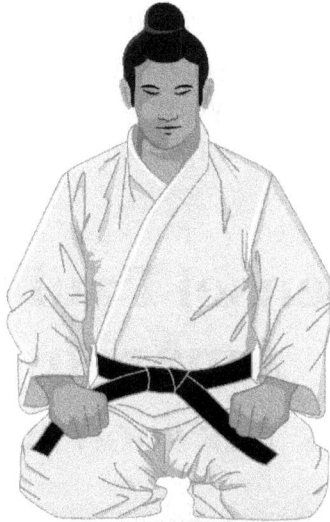

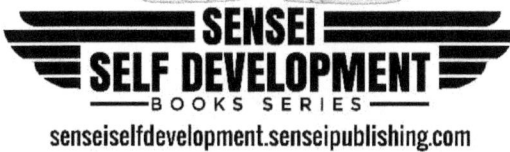

senseiselfdevelopment.senseipublishing.com

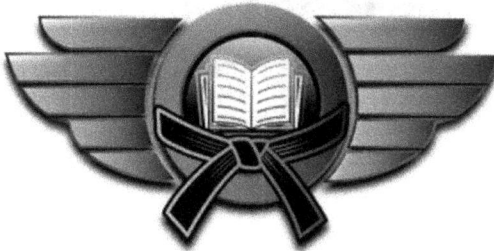

Join Our Publishing Journey!

If you would like to receive FREE BOOKS, please visit **www.senseipublishing.com**. Join our newsletter by entering your email address in the pop-up box

Follow Sensei Paul David on Amazon

CLICK THE LOGO BELOW

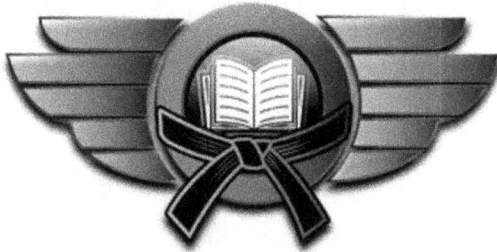

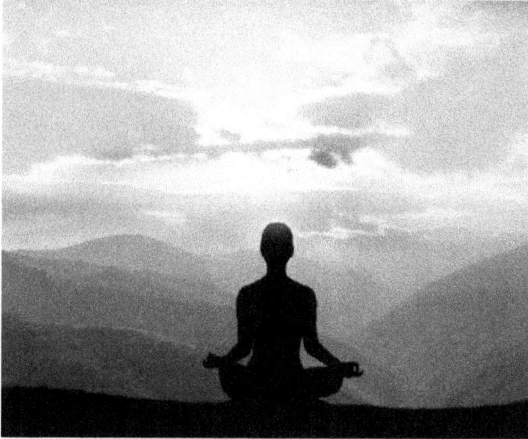

FREE BONUS!!!
Experience Over 25 FREE Engaging Guided Meditations!

Prized Skills & Practices for Adults & Kids. Help Restore Deep-Sleep, Lower Stress, Improve Posture, Navigate Uncertainty & More.

Download the Free Insight Timer App and click the link below:
http://insig.ht/sensei_paul

About Sensei Publishing

Sensei Publishing commits itself to helping people of all ages transform into better versions of themselves by providing high-quality and research-based self-development books with an emphasis on mental health and guided meditations. Sensei Publishing offers well-written e-books, audiobooks, paperbacks and online courses that simplify complicated but practical topics in line with its mission to inspire people towards positive transformation.

It's a great day to be alive!

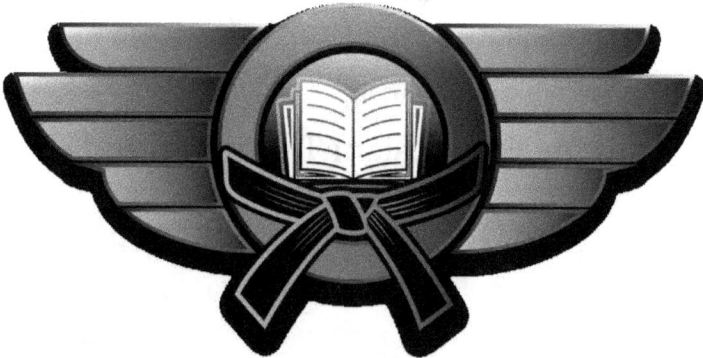

About the Author

I create simple & transformative eBooks & Guided Meditations for Adults & Children proven to help navigate uncertainty, solve niche problems & bring families closer together.

I'm a former finance project manager, private pilot, jiu-jitsu instructor, musician & former University of Toronto Fitness Trainer. I prefer a science-based approach to focus on these & other areas in my life to stay humble & hungry to evolve. I hope you enjoy my work and I'd love to hear your feedback.

- It's a great day to be alive!

Sensei Paul David

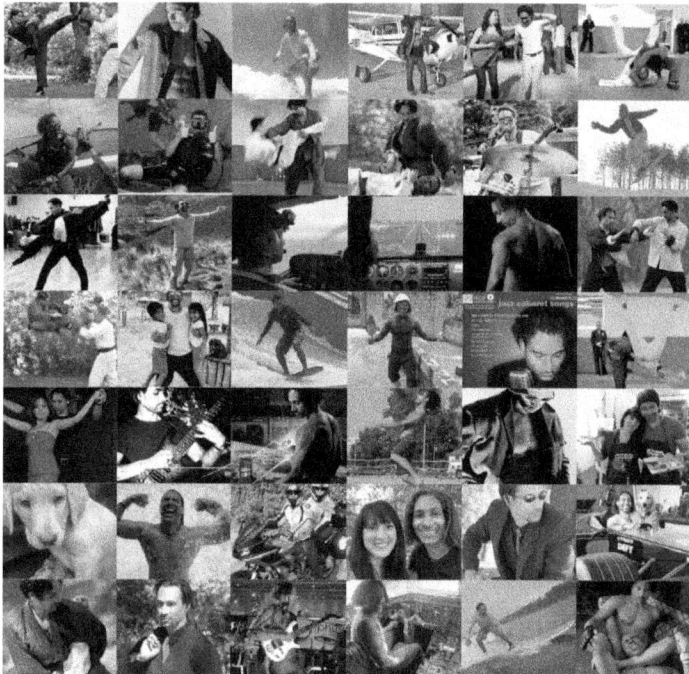

Scan & Follow/Like/Subscribe: Facebook, Instagram, YouTube: @senseipublishing

Scan using your phone/iPad camera for Social Media
Visit us at www.senseipublishing.com and sign up for our
newsletter to learn more about our exciting books and to
experience our FREE Guided Meditations for Kids & Adults.

www.ingramcontent.com/pod-product-compliance
Lightning Source LLC
Chambersburg PA
CBHW071244020426
42333CB00015B/1624